BAAR PRODUCTS, INC.
PO Box 60
Downingtown, PA 19335 USA
800-269-2502

Third Edition

ISBN 978-1508634539

Castor Oil Pack Therapy

Application & Instruction

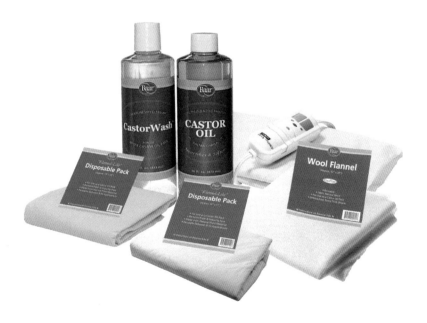

Table of Contents

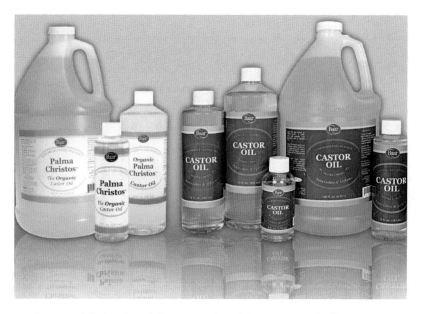

Castor Oil, both cold-pressed, cold-processed (known as Palma Christi), or **Organic** *Castor Oil (known as Palma Christos™) are used to create the Castor Oil Pack.*

Introduction to Castor Oil Pack Therapy

Castor oil is extracted from the seed of the castor oil plant named Ricinus communis. Castor oil has an extremely long and diverse history of use. In fact, castor bean seeds are believed to have been used over 4,000 years ago and have even been found in Egyptian tombs[1]. In earlier times, castor oil was referred to as "Palma Christi." This is because of the plant's palmate leaves and the oil's miraculous therapeutic properties which are reminiscent of the healing abilities of the Christ. Due to the powerful healing properties of the oil, the name "Palma Christi" stuck.

Historically, castor oil has been taken internally for its laxative effects on the body, however, its therapeutic benefits go beyond its laxative properties. This ancient oil can be used topically for immune support, skin care and muscle and joint pain relief.

The external use of castor oil is referred to as Castor Oil Pack Therapy, in which "packs" are made and applied to various parts of the body. A castor oil pack is placed on the skin to increase the body's circulation (especially the lymphatic system) and help with the functioning of tissues and organs underneath the skin. The packs are most commonly used to support digestion, improve assimilations and eliminations, and relieve and reduce inflammations in the body. Castor oil packs have been documented as a holistic approach for various issues in the body.

The benefits of the Castor Oil Pack are well defined in

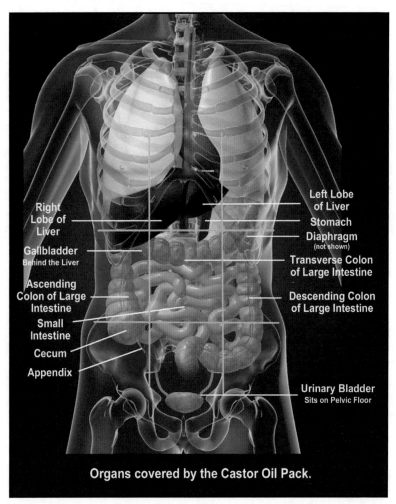

Right Lobe of Liver	Left Lobe of Liver
	Stomach
	Diaphragm (not shown)
Gallbladder Behind the Liver	
	Transverse Colon of Large Intestine
Ascending Colon of Large Intestine	Descending Colon of Large Intestine
Small Intestine	
Cecum	
Appendix	Urinary Bladder Sits on Pelvic Floor

Organs covered by the Castor Oil Pack.

the acronym CARE: Circulation, Assimilation, Relaxation, and Elimination. Without proper *circulation*, the body's ability to heal itself is severely impaired; *assimilation* is essential for digesting and absorbing food; *relaxation* is necessary for the body to self-heal; *elimination* enables the body to rid itself of toxins and cleanse the internal organs. The use of the Castor Oil Pack profoundly and positively affects each one of these processes[2].

Castor oil packs are commonly used for:
- Appendicitis
- Arthritis
- Colitis
- Congestion
- Constipation
- Digestive Complaints
- Epilepsy
- Gall Stones
- Headaches, Migraines
- Intestinal Disorders
- Immune Health
- Kidney Function
- Liver Conditions
- Lymphatic Function
- Scleroderma
- Stretch Marks
- Toxemia
- Uterine & Ovarian Cysts

The effectiveness of castor oil may be attributed to its unique chemical composition. Castor oil is packed with fatty acids. Almost 90% of the fatty acid content consists of ricinoleic acid. Such high concentrations of ricinoleic acid may be the reason for the healing properties of castor oil.

A double blind study conducted with healthy volunteer subjects demonstrated an increase in lymphocytes specifically the level of activity of T-cell lymphocytes in the group that used castor oil packs. These T-cells originate from bone marrow and mature in the thymus gland. They work to kill various molds, viruses, yeasts and bacteria. T-11 cell lymphocytes supply a fundamental antibody which keeps the body's defense system strong[3].

Castor oil works by penetrating deep into the skin's surface and targeting underlying areas. Once penetrated into the skin, the oil stimulates circulation and works to detoxify, enhancing the body's natural healing processes.

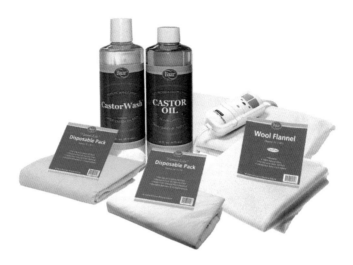

Castor Oil Pack Therapy: A Step-by-Step Guide

Castor oil packs may be applied to various areas of the body. They are most commonly placed over the abdomen area, targeting the liver and organs that support proper eliminations and detoxification in the body. The majority of the liver is located toward the right front side of the body so you will want to make sure this area is covered by the pack. The pack should extend from the lower portion of the rib cage to the upper edge of the hipbone. It should cover the entire abdomen, extending from side to side.

The best time to use a castor oil pack is in the evening or when you are able to fully rest and relax without interruption. It is an ideal time for reading inspirational material or listening to calming music or simply connecting with your inner self.

Before you begin, decide where you are going to set-up

the therapy; most people choose a bed or a sofa. Lay out an old sheet, towel or Large Disposable Pack (#755) to catch any castor oil that may drip from the pack.

Creating the Castor Oil Pack

The next step is actually creating the castor oil pack. Making a castor oil pack is an easy process. Throughout the years, castor oil packs have been made in various ways. All of these methods for making the pack are similar, but they have small differences according to preference. We will review two of the most popular ways to make the pack, and you can expect the same great results in either case.

You will need:

- Cold Pressed, Cold Processed Castor Oil (Product #753, #752, #751 or #750)

OR

- Palma Christos™ **Organic** Castor Oil (Product #7980, #7988 or #7981), also Cold Pressed, Cold Processed.

CLOTH OPTIONS:

- Unbleached Wool Flannel (#757) or Cotton Flannel (#759) or Large Disposable Pack (#755) or Small Disposable Pack (#799)

AND:

- King Size Electric Heating Pad (#10466)
- CastorWash™ (#769, to clean and alkalize the skin)
- Extra Disposable Pack* (#755, used to protect bedding or furniture)
- Wash cloth or sponge* (to apply the CastorWash™)

  * Optional items that you may prefer to use

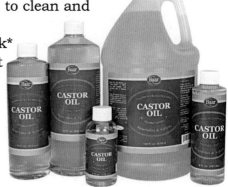

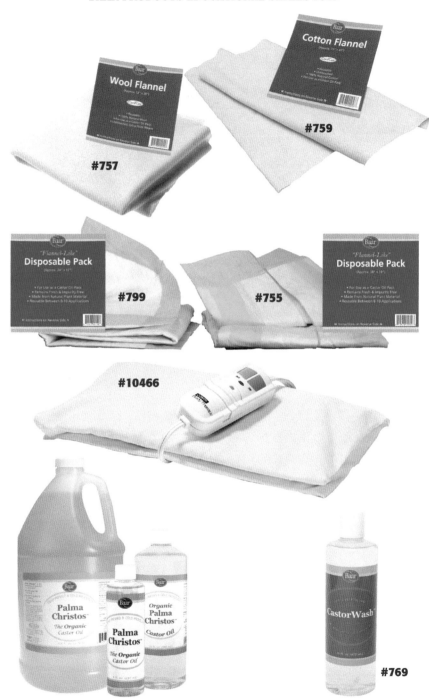

Wool Flannel

#757

Cotton Flannel

#759

"Flannel-Like" Disposable Pack

#799

#755

"Flannel-Like" Disposable Pack

#10466

Palma Christos™ The Organic Castor Oil

Organic Palma Christos™ Castor Oil

CastorWash™

#769

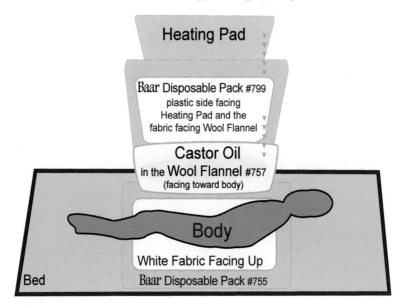

Pack Assembly

Method 1:

The first method for making the castor oil pack is a very traditional way. This pack is made with a piece of wool flannel. Wool was the original material that was suggested for use in Edgar Cayce's work, so many people like to follow this recommendation.

To make the pack:

1. Lay the Large Disposable Pack (#755) down to protect any bedding or furniture.
2. Turn your Heating Pad (#10466) to a low, medium or high setting, depending on personal comfort levels and place on the Large Disposable Pack (#755).
3. Place a 2nd smaller blue Disposable Pack (#799) on top of the Heating Pad with the plastic side against the Heating Pad (OPTIONAL: Protects your Heating Pad from oil).
4. Fold the Wool Flannel (#757) into 3 layers, creating a thick layer of wool.

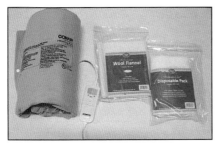

Method 1: *The first three items you will need are the Heating Pad (enclosed in a blue cover), the Wool (or Cotton) Flannel and one or two Disposable Packs.*

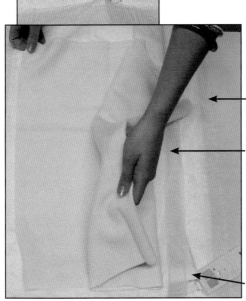

The light indicates that the Heating Pad is on and warming up.

Place a Disposable Pack <u>underneath</u> your Heating Pad to protect surfaces. Place a 2nd disposable pack <u>on top</u> of the Heating Pad with the plastic side against the Heating Pad (optional for protecting the Heating Pad). Fold your Wool or Cotton Flannel into three layers and then place on top of all.

Heating Pad

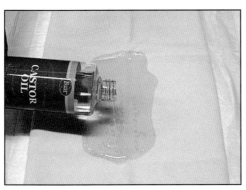

Pour 4 oz. of Castor Oil onto the wool until it is saturated but not dripping. Have this sit for about 10 minutes so the Heating Pad warms the Castor Oil.

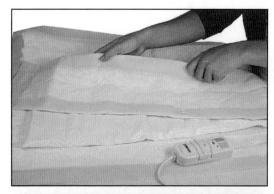

Method 2: *Use one Disposable Pack underneath your Heating Pad for protection and a second pack on top of the Heating Pad.*

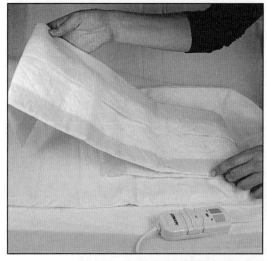

You can fold the Disposable Pack as shown to create a pocket which will hold the oil.

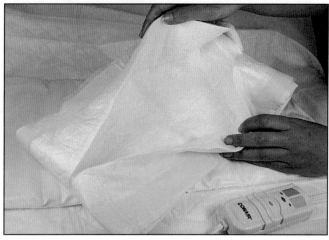

5. Place the folded Wool Flannel (#757) on top of the 2nd Disposable Pack.

6. Pour 4 oz. of Castor Oil (#753, #752, #751 or #750) or Palma Christos™ **Organic** Castor Oil (#7980, #7988 or #7981) onto the wool until it is saturated but not dripping.

7. Allow saturated wool to sit for about 10 minutes on the Heating Pad so it will warm the Castor Oil. Test oil temperature before applying to body.

** Cotton Flannel (#759) is also available to use in place of Wool Flannel. It is an excellent alternative for anyone with a sensitivity or allergy to wool.

Pack Assembly

Method 2:

The second option uses a Baar Disposable Pack as a substitute for Wool or Cotton Flannel. This is also a great option for those with a sensitivity to wool. The Disposable Pack consists of an all natural, "flannel-like" material, which is absorbent on one side and coated with a plastic covering on the other side to protect the Heating Pad. The Disposable Pack is a very convenient option because it tends to be less messy. It may also be used underneath the body to protect the area you are resting on. This method is a much quicker way to make a pack and is easy to use when traveling.

To make the pack:

1. Lay the Large Disposable Pack (#755) down to protect bedding or furniture (green side down, white up).

2. Place the Heating Pad (#10466) on top of the Disposable Pack and turn your Heating Pad to a low, medium or high setting.

3. Place a second Disposable Pack (#799 or #755) on top of the Heating Pad with the plastic side against the Heating Pad.

4. Pour about 4 oz. of Castor Oil (#753, #752, #751 or #750) or Palma Christos™ **Organic** Castor Oil (#7980, #7988 or #7981) onto the Disposable Pack on top of

the Heating Pad until the Pack is saturated but not dripping.

5. Allow the saturated Pack to sit for about 10 minutes on the Heating Pad so it will warm the Castor Oil.

Applying the Pack to Your Skin

Now that your pack is made all you need to do is apply it to the skin. Once the pack is warm, lie down on the bed or sofa that you've chosen for your therapy. Flip the pack with Heating Pad onto your abdomen or desired area (so that the Castor Oil is against the skin).

Leave the pack on for about 1 to 2 hours. According to the severity of the condition, you may leave the pack on longer. If the pack feels uncomfortable in temperature, you may turn the heat up or down according to your preference.

> **Do not** apply heat if you are experiencing severe abdominal pain.
> Apply pack **without heat.** See page 16.
> **Do not** warm the pack in the oven or microwave.

After You Finish Using the Pack

When you finish your therapy, turn the Heating Pad off and put it to the side. Remove the pack with Castor Oil and fold it in half. Store the pack in a leak-proof container or a plastic bag. Keep the pack in a cool, dark area, preferably the refrigerator. Packs may be used repeatedly by replenishing them with Castor Oil before each use. When stored correctly, the Wool and Cotton Flannel packs usually last for about 1½ to 2 months and the Disposable Packs last 8 to 10 applications. If the pack becomes discolored or starts to smell differently, dispose of it and make a new pack.

Use the CastorWash (Product #769) to cleanse the skin after using the pack. This helps with alkalizing the area and removing toxins left on the skin's surface. The CastorWash helps remove the Castor Oil from the skin quickly and easily.

Safe Storage for Your Castor Oil Pack

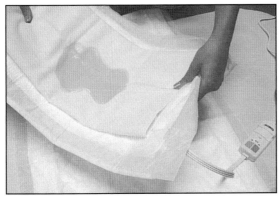

One method of storage is folding both the Flannel and the Disposable Pack together. Fold toward the middle so that the Castor Oil is contained by the Flannel.

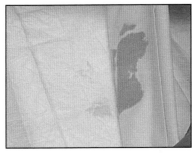

You may also store the Flannel and the Disposable Packs separately.

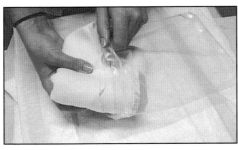

Fold the wool so it will store in a plastic bag.

And then fold the Disposable Pack and place in its own plastic bag.

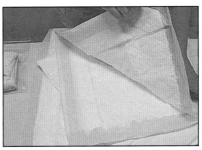

Deciding How Often to Repeat Pack Therapy

Castor Oil Packs should be done in cycles. It is generally recommended that the pack be applied 3 to 7 times a week for best results. For most applications, use the pack for at least 3 days in a row. Then you may want to take a few days off from using it. Your health condition and the severity of that condition will determine how often you will want to use the Castor Oil Pack. Consult with your health care practitioner.

A Therapy Recommended by Medical Doctors, Naturopaths, Osteopaths and Edgar Cayce

Castor oil pack therapy has been used throughout the decades for many different ailments. Most people are familiar with the therapy because of Edgar Cayce, known as "The Sleeping Prophet." Cayce was a renowned medical intuitive in the early to mid-1900s. There are countless readings in which he recommended castor oil packs for immune system enhancement as well as other conditions. There are also reports from his patients who have explained the successes they've had. (See "Feedback and Testimonials" on page 21.)

Many people still follow Cayce's recommendations today and report wonderful results. Because so many people find value with this alternative therapy, the medical community is beginning to recognize the benefits of castor oil pack therapy as well.

Gladys McGarey, M.D., M.D.(H)

Dr. Gladys Taylor McGarey is internationally known for her pioneering work in holistic medicine, the physician-patient partnership and natural birthing. She has practiced medicine for 50 years and has advocated a holistic approach to patient care through her worldwide lectures and writing. In 1992, she was one of 100 physicians and researchers appointed to the National Institutes of Health's (NIH) newly created Office of Alternative Medicine. A founding member and past president of the American Holistic medical Association, past president of the Arizona Homeopathic Board, a director of the American Board of Holistic Medicine, Cofounder and lead physician of the ARE Clinic from 1968-1989, Cofounder of the Academy of Parapsychology and Medicine, Cofounder of The Scottsdale Holistic Medical Group, and Creator and president of The Foundation for Living Medicine.[4]

Treatment for Pregnancy Issues and Menstrual Pain

I have used Castor oil for myself and patients for the past 50 years. I have used it as a pack, without heat, for threatened miscarriages, abdominal and back discomfort during pregnancies, and any other time that a pregnant woman chooses to use it. With heat, it helps menstrual pain and can be placed on the part of the body where the pain is greatest.

Benefits of Castor Oil

Let us not forget the Castor Oil Pack! Place it over the upper right side of your abdomen. It can be used with heat for 60 to 90 minutes any time of day and before bedtime. If time does not allow the hour before bedtime, it can be used without heat, and you can sleep with it for several hours or all night long. It should not be used with heat any time an inflammatory process is involved. When you put it on, be aware it has been called the Palma Christi (the Palm of Christ). You are placing this healing, loving, quieting, divine energy over your liver and solar plexus. This is the area of the third chakra where we carry stress and judgments, as well as anger and resentment. Using the castor oil pack with its healing energy over this area allows us to move into a space of divine peace, and sleep comes more readily.

One of the reasons castor oil is so effective in the healing process is that it is absorbed by the lymphatics of the skin, and carried to the deeper lymphatics, helping to keep the lymph clean. It is like rain in the mountains. The rain comes down between the rocks, goes into little rivulets, and then into pools, transferring into larger streams, rivers and, ultimately, out into the ocean. The lymphatic system is like that, and castor oil helps keep the lymph clean. So whatever else castor oil does, it certainly serves a vital role in the cleansing process associated with the lymphatic system.

Castor oil helps ease lymphatic congestion, venus stasis, muscle tension and inflammation. In my experience, women who have used the castor oil pack for small uterine fibroids frequently have been able to eliminate them completely, and some ovarian cysts have responded well to the castor oil pack.[5]

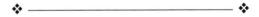

Christiane Northrup, M.D.

Treatment and Prevention of Cramps
Lying down with a castor oil pack on your lower abdomen for sixty minutes two to four times per week is often very helpful for both treatment and prevention of cramps and pelvic pain. Edgar Cayce, the renowned medical intuitive of the early to mid-1900s, recommended this immune-system-enhancing treatment for all kinds of conditions. *Note: Do not use these if they increase your pain or if you are bleeding heavily.*[6]

Minor Breast Inflammation
Put the cloth on the breast, cover with plastic, and then apply the heating pad. Turn the setting on the pad up to moderate, and then hot, if you can stand it. Leave it on for an hour.[7]

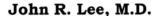

John R. Lee, M.D.

What to Do for Healing the Uterus/Fibroids

Eat a plant-based, fiber-rich diet (at least 20-30 g fiber per day).

Take a liver-supporting and detoxifying herbal formula that includes some or all of the following herbs: *Bupleurum*, milk thistle, barberry or goldenseal, burdock root, yellow dock, dandelion root.

Take a uterus-healing herbal formula that includes some or all of the following herbs: myrrh, red raspberry, cayenne, *Bupleurum*, yarrow, vitex and lady's mantle.

Use a castor oil pack 2 to 4 times a week.[8]

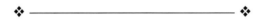

Harold J. Reilly, D.Ph.T., D.S.

Colonics, together with castor oil packs and manipulation, are truly the distinctive hallmark of the Cayce drugless therapy. Certainly in my own practice and experience they have produced some of the most dramatic and fantastic healing results.

I have found the castor oil packs to be invaluable in all cases of constipation, a variety of gallbladder, kidney, and liver disorders, pelvic disorders, inflammation, gallstones, and kidney stones.

For home use I would advise the castor-oil packs for chronic constipation, gallbladder trouble, sluggish liver, and many types of abdominal conditions, but check with your doctor first, for discomfort or pain may be the symptom of a serious ailment.[9]

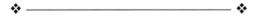

John O.A. Pagano, D.C.

Liver Support

Another effective procedure I suggest to some patients is

the application of warm castor oil packs directly over the liver. The simplest way to accomplish this is to saturate the liver area with castor oil; place a warm, damp, soft cloth (preferably white flannel, four layers thick) over the area; then cover with a piece of plastic wrap. A heating pad, set at medium, is placed over the entire pack for one to two hours. I have found, to my satisfaction, that massaging the liver or applying hot castor oil packs to it are among the healthiest measures that can be taken to help this organ perform its function of purifying the blood.[10]

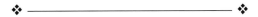

Linda Caputi, R.N.

Breaking up Lesions and Adhesions

Hot castor oil packs were usually given in a three-day series and were kept on for from one to three hours over the entire right abdomen, both anterior and posterior from the right costal margin to the crest of the ileum and covering the area of the caecum and umbilicus. These hot packs were said to start the breakup of the lacteal lesions and adhesions. The heat alone would certainlhy tend to increase the circulation of the area. it was also implied that the castor oil itself would have a beneficial effect by absorption through the skin. In many cases a period of abdominal massage and kneading of the right side of the abdomen was instructed immediately after the removal of the packs, to help in the break-up of the lesions and adhesions.[11]

Applications Suggestions

Persistency and consistency are called for with chronic conditions. You can use the pack for 3 days in a row, take a break for 4 days, and then repeat. This is a typical series of castor oil packs but many other variations were given (4 days on - 3 days off, or 5 days on - 2 days off, every other day, etc.)[12]

Feedback and Testimonials

Customer Feedback

The following are comments from customers who have used Castor Oil Pack Therapy for the successful relief of a variety of common ailments.

* Excerpts from the Archives of Baar Products, Inc.

† Excerpts from the A.R.E. Journal and written by William McGarey, M.D. (Date & Volume is noted after each excerpt.)

"I love your products — Castor Oil Packs are wonderful. I have used them for all kinds of ailments for me, my family and my employees."

[*© 2013 Baar Products, Inc., Case #68258, J.L., Beaverton, OR]

"FINALLY I've found this product exactly as it is worded (cold processed cold pressed Castor oil) and at the quantity I needed and price I could afford!! Thanks ever so much!"

[*© 2013 Baar Products, Inc., Case # 170019, C.W., Parma, OH]

"Castor Oil will at times help when other therapies are ineffective."

[*© 2013 Baar Products, Inc., Case #190560, A.J., MD.,WV]

This is a very good item. I started getting into alternative medicine and Castor oil is good for a lot of health issues. This kit supplies everything needed.

[*© 2013 Baar Products, Inc., Case #169267, V.W. Gaithersburg, MD]

Castor Oil Packs have helped me sooo much. I've been putting them everywhere, on my knees and on my back, and I think it really helped me.

[*© 2013 Baar Products, Inc., Case #164136, P.C., New Bern, NC]

I can't say enough what your product Castor oil has done for me and my clients and friends, it is a healing product. I am a licensed massage therapist in NC and I will continue to use this and more of your products.

[*© 2013 Baar Products, Inc., Case #100616, D.B., Wilson, N.C.]

Alcoholism

An alcoholic for more than 20 years is the description one of our correspondents gave herself in a research report which she submitted recently. But she used castor oil packs on her abdomen for an entirely different reason four years ago. It seemed that she had developed a severe abdominal pain. She did not consult her doctor, so her own diagnosis of "probably an intestinal disorder" will have to suffice, no matter how inadequate. She reports that her pain lessened a little each day, as she applied the packs on a twice daily routine. An apparent constipation was thoroughly corrected on the second day, but she continued the packs for a period of two weeks.

The most remarkable result of her own little adventure in consciousness, however, is the real point of this story. She adds as a postscript to her report that "Since the day I first used oil packs, I have not touched a drop of liquor - nor have I had the desire to do so. I was an alcoholic for more than 20 years. I used to drink myself to sleep every single night."

My question is: What is it that happens to people that makes a simple act of healing turn their lives into a new channel of living? Why should applications of castor oil packs rival Alcoholics Anonymous in this particular event in time and space? Life offers us a multitude of unanswered questions, doesn't it?

[† November, 1975, Volume 10, No. 6, page 276, Copyright © 1975 by the

Edgar Cayce Foundation, Virginia Beach, VA.]

Ankle Injuries

I have seen castor oil packs placed around an injured ankle relieve pain that had persisted for days after the repair of a laceration. Thus it was not with a great deal of surprise that I read the results of therapy applied by one A.R.E. member to her child. Isaac (Mrs. Bell's tree-climbing-aged son) fell fifteen feet from a tree he had almost conquered and struck the ground with his hip. His family doctor recommended hot tub soaks; and his mother supplemented the treatment with one of the Cayce remedies for muscular sprains. However, repeated efforts in this direction brought only swollen tissues. The following afternoon, and again that night, a castor oil pack was applied with a heating pad; the next morning Isaac was up and ready for Monday morning school. There was no swelling and very little tenderness. After school the tenderness was gone, and Isaac had forgotten that he had failed in his effort to fly.

[† November, 1976, Volume 11, No. 6, page 272, Copyright © 1976 by the Edgar Cayce Foundation, Virginia Beach, VA.]

Appendix

"My first contact with you was when I had an appendix attack and I was told by the doctors the next attack would result in surgery. I took time off from work and did castor oil pack for 3 days. That was the last time my appendix drew attention."

[*© 2013 Baar Products, Inc., Case # 170570, L.D., Santee, CA.]

Bed Down with Castor Oil

Castor Oil stories continue to be an almost daily occurrence in our experience. One of our patients who has used castor oil packs rather extensively became concerned about his landlord, who is a widower and who was diagnosed after a stroke as having high blood pressure and a large abdominal aortic aneurysm. He was in constant pain from it, and the medicines he obtained from the medical center where he was treated only seemed to make him worse. The advocate of castor oil packs finally convinced his friend to try using the packs on his abdomen in spite of the fact that the landlord couldn't understand how in the world something like that would have any effect.

After less than a week of using the packs, the pain had subsided so much that the landlord waxed enthusiastic. He waxed so much, in fact, that he started buying castor oil by the gallon. He purchased several yards of wool flannel and rigged up his bed like no prescription I have ever given. Over the mattress cover, he placed a large plastic cover. Then came several layers of flannel - then two more layers of flannel, then a blanket on top of that. The room was always heated, even while the landlord slept. Then he poured castor oil on the flannel over the entire bed and climbed in between the several layers of wool flannel. Every day he would add some castor oil to the bed, and apparently when the whole setup became too old to be of value, he would discard the blanket, the flannel, etc., and bring in some new materials.

The story would just be humorous - even if true, which it is - if he derived no significant benefits from the treatments. He didn't even wipe off the oil from the skin when he got up in the morning. Truly a monumental experiment for one man. But the experimenter still continues to see his doctor regularly, tells him what he is doing, and feels better than he has in years. Now he is able to do his gardening, do the carpentering needed around his place, and recently even climbed up on the roof to fix a leak. His physical condition is better; his blood pressure apparently is improved; and he has a new life in front of him.

He did his own personal research project after reading much about the use of castor oil as given in the Cayce readings in the booklet, Edgar Cayce and the Palma Christi. Healings of the body indeed may come about in many ways and manners.

[† November, 1975, Volume 10, No. 6, page 275, Copyright © 1975 by the Edgar Cayce Foundation, Virginia Beach, VA.]

Bee Sting and Arthritis

Stephen Hasman tells the story of his brother being stung by a bee in Ohio. He came into the house with "goose bumps" on his arm, the evidence of the bee sting showing clearly. It was already sore and the swelling had become markedly evident. Stephen, who has had much experience with castor oil, got out his bottle and placed just one drop "on the welt which had an open puncture on it." In less than ten minutes, his brother reported that the soreness had gone and the swelling for the most part had subsided. After supper, there were no complaints. His brother's wife was asked why they didn't have castor oil in their home.

From Kentucky comes another report dealing with this same oil being used for arthritis:

"Since the early 1970s when I first obtained your book, Edgar Cayce and the Palma Christi, I have been experimenting with castor oil. I have also been reading The A.R.E. *Journal* to see if my results are the same as others.

"My brother-in-law was scheduled for an operation on his finger (the one next to his forefinger) to scrape off the crystals that had formed there and that were giving him a lot of pain. His mother suggested he check with me on the castor oil, and I told him I didn't think it would help as the finger was really in bad shape. However, as it turned out, he had quite a herd of cattle and was unable to have the operation as scheduled, so used the castor oil anyway - just rubbed it on, he said. Two weeks later he visited his doctor who told him, 'Well, it's gone.'"

Another story from the same source:

"I have a lady friend and neighbor in her late 80s who called me one day. The two middle fingers of her hand were locked and had been for years. Her thumb was twice its regular size, and the little finger and forefinger were giving her so much pain she was crying and couldn't use them. I stressed to her that it would not be possible to unlock the fingers or correct the thumb, but based on the results of my brother-in-law, we might be able to save the other two fingers - or at least stop the pain. She didn't have a bathtub, so we got a container for a foot bath and used a pound or so of Epsom salts in which I asked her to bathe her feet for half an hour each evening, all the time pressing, rubbing or flexing her feet (simply to keep her hands in the solution). I told her then to wrap the hands in castor oil for the evening and place a castor oil pack on her stomach with a heating pad. She called a couple of days later saying that the fingers had stopped paining and she was continuing treatment.

"I know a couple of other people who were bothered with crystals, so I thought it would be interesting to take a picture of her hands since no one would believe it without the pictures. So I borrowed a camera and went over no later than two weeks after she had started treatments. To my immense surprise, she had those two fingers unlocked and was making a quilt. She said she used the foot bath with water as hot as she could stand it for the time I stressed, then put the castor oil pack on her stomach with a heating pad and wrapped her hands with castor oil cloths, put on rubber gloves, took her magnifying glass and a book to bed with her and alternated her hands on the heating pad the rest of the evening. No pain in the other fingers, thumb greatly improved, fingers still working okay and she still works on the quilting. Whenever they begin to ache, she just gives them a repeat treatment."

Quite amazing, isn't it? Some of these stories definitely touch new areas in healing.

[† November, 1982, Volume 17, No. 6, page 279, Copyright © 1982 by the Edgar Cayce Foundation, Virginia Beach, VA.]

Castor Oil and Cancer Pain

Pain in the terminal cancer patient is perhaps the most feared complication of neoplastic diseases in the human being. One wonders where the pain actually originates-for pain is perhaps the most difficult symptom to pin down and the least understood. Methods of cancer therapy derived from unorthodox sources seem to produce some help in this direction. In my own experience with cancer patients who were too far advanced with the disease to be helped by any of the therapies available, I have seen one traditional aid bring much relief from pain during the terminal days. Quite recently, a 62-year-old man developed a cancer of the brain. By the time he came under medical observation, it was quite advanced; then, a second malignancy was discovered in the wall of the bladder. Weight loss had come rapidly, and the only therapy offered him was chemotherapy. When the family consulted us, the patient was terminal, in bed and obviously had not long to go. He was advised to use castor oil packs on the abdomen. He had not used any pain medication up to that point, and remained pain-free until twenty-four hours before he passed away. Then he developed some pain in one flank. The castor oil pack was applied locally there, too, and he became comfortable once again.

An earlier instance of the use of these packs came nearly twenty years ago, when I was called upon to care for a woman who had a large abdominal cancer which was far advanced when I first saw her. She had become unable to care for herself. She refused surgery of any kind and went into a rest home, since she had no living relatives. There she received coffee enemas and abdominal castor oil packs daily for the next forty days, until her death. She had no pain at any time. One wonders if these cases - and I'm sure I am not alone in observing this - are simply coincidences, or does a soothing application with particular vibrations bring about a reaction in the autonomic nervous system of the lymphatic system which eliminates the situation that causes pain? At times there seem to be more cases that deviate from the rule than there are ones that obey it.

[† May, 1976, Volume 11, No. 3, page 137, Copyright © 1976 by the Edgar Cayce Foundation, Virginia Beach, VA.]

Concrete Example of Castor Oil Use

Mabel Alford related a castor oil story during our week's program on Home and Marriage in Virginia Beach last year. A longtime A.R.E. member, she has attended many workshops and read widely in the Cayce material. Though she is experienced in taking care of herself, this time she forgot for a while. About a year ago, she was mixing up cement and neglected to put gloves on, thinking that it was not really necessary. No problem doing the work that morning, but later on in the afternoon, her hands started to hurt. As the pain grew more severe, the skin started to peel off in places. She took some aspirin that night, but couldn't sleep because of the pain. She tried soaking her hands in aspirin water, but that didn't help. Finally, in the wee hours of the morning, she remembered castor oil. She actually dipped her hands in the oil, put on stocking gloves and then, when she got back into bed, slept like a baby.

Prior to using the castor oil, her hands were stiff and the tissues edematous, and she had visions of not being able to work the next week. (She is a check-out clerk at a supermarket.) But when she took the gloves off the next morning, there was no pain, no swelling, and she found no problems in using her fingers and hands at work.

[† September, 1975, Volume 10, No. 5, page 223, Copyright © 1975 by the Edgar Cayce Foundation, Virginia Beach, VA.]

Detoxify

"So much healing, so many doctors, I have the opportunity to detoxify before next labs. I blew the doctors away with my liver results. Castor Oil packs work. I am called an enigma. I tried to tell them what I was doing along with their assistance. I got the, 'not possible response.' Yet they do not have answers to their questions. So I will continue to stay on my feet and watch them scratch their heads wondering what they missed. Thank you again."

[*© 2014 Baar Products, Inc., Case #210210, J.K., MA]

Finger Injury

Healing is everybody's business or, at least, so thought the ten-year-old son of a laboratory technician, who corresponds with us. This is the story again of castor oil. It seems that Mike is the center on their football squad, and he really loves to play. His brother accidentally dealt him a low blow when he slammed a truck door shut on the index and middle fingers of Mike's right hand. Mike had a most important football game scheduled six days later, and his right hand plays a vital part in such a contest. His mother continues the story:

"At the hospital, his hand was splinted and we were told he would not be able to participate in sports for three weeks at the earliest. Mike insisted that he use the castor oil packs 24 hours after the injury. The fingers were cut and had some infection in them. That boy soaked his own fingers in warm water for 20 minutes and applied the castor oil therapy himself. I returned from night school and he told me what he had done. He continued his own treatment for three more days and he played in that important football game. I had taped his fingers for protection, but no splints were allowed. By the following week, he was completely healed. I never thought his fingers would look right again - but today they are as if they had never been injured."

[† November, 1976, Volume 6, No. 2, page 272, Copyright © 1976 by the Edgar Cayce Foundation, Virginia Beach, VA.]

Fingers and Castor Oil

The healing influence of the oil of the Ricinus communis has been documented thousands of times now, and the following stories just amplify the documentation.

Swelling of the left middle finger between the interphalangeal joints bothered Edna Atkins, but she fussed along with the swelling for many weeks before actually getting down to the business of treating the finger. She had heard how good castor oil was for a variety of ailments but had just never tried it. She related the following: "I finally got out some oil one evening while watching TV and just rubbed it around the second joint a while. I did this two evenings, leaving it on when I went to bed. The third night I was again going to rub the joint, but could not find the spot any longer. I couldn't even be sure which hand or finger it was, as there was no sign of swelling or difference between any fingers any longer!" She didn't even know the diagnosis, but the cure was great!

[† November, 1981, Volume 16, No. 7, page 287, Copyright © 1981 by the Edgar Cayce Foundation, Virginia Beach, VA.]

Gall Stones

"I am so grateful that my gallstones are gone and that I did not have to have the surgery I dreaded. I certainly want to add my name to the list of people who got relief from using this alternative treatment. I also want to say that I continue to use castor oil packs for other discomforts like indigestion, GERD and muscle spasms. It continues to bring relief, and just the heating pad alone does NOT bring the same results."

The Miracle Oil, by David E. Kukor[13]

Knee Pain

I am not sure whether the following story has a near relative in the Cayce data or if it was simply an adaptation of a specific therapy treatment. The story comes from Esther Spearrin, who has attended A.R.E. conferences at Seabeck (near Seattle) for many years:

"I had my knee operated on after an injury and, because a piece of the bone was broken right at the knee joint, surgery was done to 'hold the piece from falling into the knee joint.' According to my orthopedic doctor, I had one bolt, two pins and wires inserted into my leg just at the knee joint or just above the knee joint to hold these together while they healed. They healed well and there was no trouble until I came to Seabeck in 1974. Then I noticed that the knee began hurting so that I could not walk upstairs without pain. I had debated before about buying a gallon of castor oil to use in packs, etc. Now I had to do so. After purchasing the oil I applied a cloth saturated with the castor oil over my knee, put plastic over that, and then a dry cloth wrapped around the knee to keep it in place overnight. I did this just a couple of times, and the rest of the week at Seabeck I had no trouble. Even now, after several years, no more difficulty has been experienced with the injury of the knee."

[† March, 1980, Volume 15, No. 2, page 49, Copyright © 1980 by the Edgar Cayce Foundation, Virginia Beach, VA.]

I have been using the castor oil packs on a knee which really helps. I was in a bicycle accident a year ago and it helped the recovery of these injuries a great deal.

[*, © 2013 Baar Products, Inc., - Case #51243, G.J., Webster City, IA, 9/28/09]

I have had three knee operations, none to replace a knee, but to replace torn ligaments (ACL) and meniscus. Each time the recovery has been tough and had taken months of therapy. Even though I have kept up with strength and stretching exercises, including yoga, I still experience pain and fatigue in my knees. I have found that placing a Castor Oil Pack around the knee, surrounded by the heating pad, then kept in place by an elastic medical wrap, does more help than any pain relief pill. I will keep these packs on for at least an hour, and I can sleep in this – with or without a heating pad – and my knee feels strong and supple the next day. I highly recommend this to anyone that mentions knee pain. I consider my legs very important these days, and treat them as such – I think they are stronger than ever and will continue to use Castor Oil Packs to keep them this way.

[*, © 2013 Baar Products, Inc., Case #338700, L.N., Downingtown, PA]

Mole

I had a puffy mole on my cheek. Every night I massaged Castor Oil into it, and the mole started to flake off! It was a natural way of removing it, and I didn't have to go to a surgeon or anything to remove it. It's gone completely now and no scar! My neighbor has done it too!

[*© 2013 Baar Products, Inc., Case #124008, K.F., Williamsburg, VA]

Mono

My daughter, who's in high school, had Mono. I had her use Castor Oil Packs (with wool) and within two weeks, she was all better! It was wonderful!

[*© 2013 Baar Products, Inc., Case #124008, K.F., VA]

Packs for the Back

A low back problem of 40 years' standing was aggravated when a patient lifted a box of rocks. She went to her doctor and received some manipulative relief. She continues: "but by November the pain had not left - in fact was getting worse. I would have to wake up in order to turn over in bed - with the help of my hands. Sitting was always painful - especially riding in a car. I decided to use the castor oil pack with the hreating pad, which I did for one to three hours every night for a week. By the end of the week, the pain was gone and has never returned. The castor oil left me wondrously pain-free and flexible for the first time in years."

[† May, 1975, Volume 10, No. 3, page 131, Copyright © 1975 by the Edgar Cayce Foundation, Virginia Beach, VA.]

Sialadenitis

On Wednesday, April 11, 2001 I saw my ear, nose, and throat doctor for the last time. I was discharged after showing him and others how I overcame Sialadenitis which leads to Sjogren's Syndrome.

Many years ago, I started getting sharp tingling sensations in the upper corners of my mouth when eating.

Then, about July 2000 lumps were showing up in my right cheek. I kept consulting dentists as I thought this was a result of ill-fitting dentures.

From dentists to dental surgeons, they wouldn't tackle my problem. Finally, a personal friend who used to teach Clinical Diagnosis and is also a Chiropractor, stated that I have Sialadenitis. He said it was calcification of the parotid glands. I was getting blockage of my salivary glands. When this happened, under my right ear, an area the size of a golf ball would swell up when I ate because of the blockage. It was often very painful.

A Tucson, AZ M.D. specializing in ear, nose, and throat treated me with Clindamycin HCL150 mg. I took 2 capsules 4 times daily for 21 days. I did this for 2 more 3 week periods. The infection didn't go away. Then another doctor friend, who by the way is also a Chiropractor, told me to try using castor oil.

Two days later (on a Saturday I shall never forget) I was at the Warehouse Vitamins Store in Tucson on West Ina Rd. The manager mentioned to me about the Edgar Cayce method of treatment and the book and the castor oil.

I couldn't wait to try it out and for the next four nights I filled a hot water bottle with boiling water. I wrapped a towel around it and laid it on my pillow. I took a second hand towel and folding it double, laid it over the other towel wrapped hot water bottle on my pillow. Then I took a washcloth and poured castor oil over it, smeared it across with my fingers and laid it on the right side of my face, under the right ear, under the right jaw.

Then I laid down on it for two hours every night for 4 nights, skipped the next 3 days, then 4 more nights and 3 passing days. As I started the 3rd week, I used too hot a water bottle burning my right cheek and under my chin. I decided to stop for a while because of the burns (they went away in a week) and noticed the rocks in my cheeks were gone. The soreness by my left ear and under it ... gone. That was a month ago and all of the problems have almost totally disappeared.

I still get that old sharp or tart feelings in the corners of my mouth but only on rare occasions.

My doctor examined me on April 12, 2001 putting his fingers in my mouth to see if any stones were present and found none.

Now as I'm writing this a week later, the dryness of the mouth has also gone.

I have told three other families who have suffered with this problem and were operated on. One man had to have the swellings drained three times. I've referred all of these families to the Cayce book and am now trying other remedies.

All I can say now is thank you. If it worked for me it could work for others so I'm making copies of this letter and sending it to Bard Lindemer in the newspaper; probably the association of Dr's who specialize in ear, nose, and throat.

[*© 2013 Baar Products, Inc., Case #23523, J.P, Tucson, AZ]

Sciatica

Thank you for the Castor Oil pack info, I have a flare up of the Sciatica spasms, and the Castor oil pack has helped me these last three days.

[*© 2013 Baar Products, Inc., Case #121287, T.G., Whittier, CA, 08/4/09]

Snoring

Experiences people have had with the oil of the Palma Christi - or castor oil - are always interesting and informative, and continue to provide us with more insights into how the body really does heal itself. From a Study Group member in California comes an account of a unique application of castor oil packs. Melodie's parents had a large degree of difficulty centering around the snoring of the male member of the species. It seems that everything had been tried. Her parents had even gone to separate rooms so that sleeping would be better. But this is her story:

"My parents are both sleeping better now, thanks to the castor oil pack. My mother has insisted that my dad wear a pack every night for the last two weeks (pack with heating pad 1 hour - then just the pack all night).

"Now instead of her being kept awake by loud, guttural, choking snores and frequent angry outcries/yelling originating from nightly dreams of fighting, she is occasionally awakened by the most soft, whimsical giggling coming from the original offender - my dad! And the snoring has ceased totally! Mom also reports an enhanced sense of humor, a very affectionate husband and a spirit of cooperation that just won't quit."

[† November, 1983, Volume 18, No. 6, page 262, Copyright © 1983 by the Edgar Cayce Foundation, Virginia Beach, VA.]

Ulcers

My Ulcer Colitis had not responded to AMA medicines. They actually made me sicker. With the blessing of my gastroenterologist, I began the castor oil protocol. I have been using the castor oil pack with phenomenal success.

[*© 2013 Baar Products, Inc., Case #153395, M.N., Austin, TX]

The following accounts, written by William McGarey, M.D., are excerpted from various issues of The Association for Research & Enlightenment (A.R.E.) Journal. All material is copyrighted by the Edgar Cayce Foundation, Virginia Beach, VA.[14]

An enthusiastic reader of the Bulletin was injured in an automobile accident, with a possible rupture of the spleen. Castor oil packs for four days brought a report from the doctor, who told her to "keep on with whatever it is you're doing ... it's working!" She tells of unlikely uses for castor oil, applied locally, to treat chest colds, ear infections, and baldness(!) She has used the castor oil packs in her family for migraine headaches, which is one of the uses Cayce actually did mention in the readings.

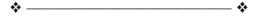

Isaac (Mrs. Bell's tree-climbing-aged son) fell fifteen feet from a tree he had almost conquered and struck the ground with his hip. His family doctor recommended hot tub soaks; and his mother supplemented the treatment with one of the Cayce remedies for muscular sprains. However, repeated efforts in this direction brought only swollen tissues. The following afternoon, and again that night, a castor oil pack was applied with a heating pad; the next morning Isaac was up and ready for Monday morning school. There was no swelling and very little tenderness. After school the tenderness was gone, and Isaac had forgotten that he had failed in his effort to fly.

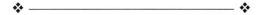

Shortly after my initial introduction to Edgar Cayce, during a weekend visit to my folks, the subject of home remedies, and castor oil in particular, emerged. I made no comment about my use of it, but rather pressed my dad, who reported that as a youth (50 or so years ago) he and his family applied it to a bleeding wart on one of their mules. They kept the bottle in the barn and made the application a part of the daily chores. He said it took a long time but that the wart healed and eventually hair grew over the spot.

I have discovered that just a little castor oil, rubbed on with the finger, on a beginning pimple or small boil, prevents it from forming; or if I'm a little late in treating, it very often disappears without coming to a head and draining on the skin surface. I suggested this to my nieces, along with a better diet, and it has worked for them also.

Approximately two months ago, I crashed into some wooden bleachers while playing volleyball. Before the evening game ended, I had an egg-sized swelling on my leg, just below the knee, in addition to the surface abrasion. After bathing, I soaked four layers of flannel, approximately 4" square, and tied this in place with an old nylon stocking. Next morning - no swelling, no signs of a bruise, no pain. I removed the dressing, and by noon I felt pain. By 2 o'clock, there was renewed swelling and signs of discoloration. I hurried home after school and immediately applied another castor oil dressing. In one hour, pain and swelling were gone, despite continued use of my leg. By the next morning, only faint discoloration defined the bruise, which surrounded the impact area and also trailed downward about one inch wide along the shin bone for about four inches. I continued the dressings for the next three evenings and through the nights.

I never did get a real bruise - to the amazement of the other teachers who wouldn't believe I had used only castor oil. (Fact is, they couldn't believe I had used castor oil!) The area never swelled again. And the abrasion healed quickly.

Prevention and cure are often born of the same measures, and there is not only wisdom, but also billions of dollars in health care being weighed in the scales as we consider what the New Age medicine would consist of.

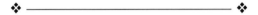

An A.R.E. member in Irvington, New Jersey, wrote that he had had palpitations of the heart which had not responded to any treatment. He used hot castor oil packs over his abdomen three days each week for an hour and a half. Every third day he took one teaspoonful of olive oil. This therapy was continued for four weeks and the symptoms cleared up for eleven months, recurring when he underwent some psychological shock. Then, after another four weeks of therapy, the symptoms disappeared again, and have been absent for over a year now.

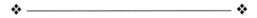

From California: "Mother had arthritis so bad she was committed to the hospital. She was there for two weeks and released with no apparent help. The arthritis was centered in her fingers which were doubled back in her palms - she didn't think she would be able to open up her fingers again. Father brought her home and started a treatment of hot castor oil - rubbing her hands, arms, and shoulders and legs three times a day. Within a period of three to four months her condition improved to the extent she could walk, use her arms, and her hands straightened out and today she is completely cured. She was 76 years old when she was at her worst and is now 81."

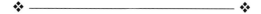

This report is from an A.R.E. member who has been working with a cooperating doctor. Her daughter, age nine, had been diagnosed as epileptic four years ago. The girl has been on Dilantin since then and complained about stomach aches, fuzziness in the right foot; she was nervous, cried often and tended toward panic in tense situations.

For two months she was given regular castor oil packs, massages, manipulations, and fairly strict dietary regimen. Her teacher said that she was "a changed person from the beginning of the year." She was considerably more relaxed and had a happy attitude; she no longer had the nightmares which once plagued her and her color was better. Her stomach aches and fuzziness in the foot were gone.

In spite of the fact that she is still on Dilantin, the changes in awareness, general health and symptomatology speak highly of what had been done for this young lady in just a period of two months. The parents are continuing with the treatments - for a long enough period of time, it is hoped, that full healing can come about.

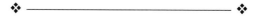

Resources

Baar Products, Inc.

Baar Products is the **Official Worldwide Exclusive Supplier of Edgar Cayce Health Care.** Baar offers a collection of natural products and remedies drawn from the work of Edgar Cayce, considered by many to be the father of modern holistic medicine.

For a complete list of Cayce-related products or to request a free catalog, call:

800-269-2502

or write: Baar Products, Inc.
PO Box 60
Downingtown, PA 19335, U.S.A.
Customer Service and International:
610-873-4591
Fax: 610-873-7945

Web: www.baar.com
Email: info@baar.com or cayce@baar.com

ARE Press: Association for Research & Enlightenment

The A.R.E. Press publishes books, videos, audiotapes, CDs, and DVDs meant to improve the quality of our readers' lives—personally, professionally, and spiritually. We hope our products support your endeavors to realize your career potential, to enhance your relationships, to improve your health, and to encourage you to make the changes necessary to live a loving, joyful, and fulfilling life.

For more information or to receive a free catalog, call:

800-333-4499

Or write: A.R.E. Press
215 67th Street
Virginia Beach, VA 25451

or email: are@EdgarCayce.org
Internet: edgarcayce.org

References

1   Grady, Harvey. *Immunomodulation Through Castor Oil Packs.* Journal of Naturopathic Medicine; Vol. 7, #1, 1999.

2   Kukor, David E. *The Miracle Oil.* Virginia Beach, VA, A.R.E. Press, 2008.

3   Grady, Harvey. *Immunomodulation Through Castor Oil Packs.* Journal of Naturopathic Medicine; Vol. 7, #1, 1999.

4   McGarey, Gladys Taylor, M.D., M.D.(H). *The Physician Within You.* Scottsdale Arizona, Inkwell Productions, 2000.

5   McGarey, Gladys Taylor., M.D., M.D. (H). *Living Medicine ~ The Dwelling Place.* Scottsdale Arizona, Inkwell Productions, 2009. Page 119.

6   Northrup, Christiane, M.D. *The Wisdom of Menopause.* New York, NY, Bantam Books, 2001. Page 244.

7   The Editors of *Prevention* Magazine Health Books. *The Doctors Book of Home Remedies.* Emmaus, PA, Rodale Press, Inc. , 1990. Page 90.

8   Lee, John R., M.D. *What Your Doctor May Not Tell You About Premenopause.* New York, NY, Warner Books, 1999. Page 103.

9   Reilly, Harold J. and Hagy Brod, Ruth. *The Edgar Cayce Handbook for Health Through Drugless Therapy.* Virginia Beach, VA, A.R.E. Press, 2008.

10 Pagano, John O.A., D.C. *Healing Psoriasis.* Hoboken, N.J., John Wiley & Sons, Inc. 2009. Page 45.

11 Caputi, Linda, R.N. *Epilepsy, Jody's Journey.* BookSurge Publishing, 2009. Page 92.

12 *ibid.* Page 197.

13 Kukor, David E. *The Miracle Oil.* Virginia Beach, VA, A.R.E. Press, 2008. Page 79.

14 McGarey, M.D., William. Various Articles. The A.R.E. Journal. ©Edgar Cayce Foundation, Virginia Beach, VA.

Dear Friends,

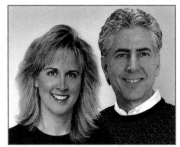

When you discover something that works well, isn't it your instinct to tell others you know about your positive experience? That's exactly how we feel about Castor Oil Pack Therapy and its powerful healing properties. For some years now, we have both used Castor Oil Packs for immune system enhancement, and at various times to help increase circulation and promote the healing of tissues, joints and ligaments.

We believe Castor Oil Pack Therapy is among the best values in the world of alternative medicine. It's been practiced successfully by people from many civilizations down through the centuries. The castor oil plant continues to be found in great abundance in nature – making this type of therapy very affordable. And, as the step-by-step instructions in this booklet will illustrate, the Castor Oil Pack is extremely easy to prepare and apply.

While we certainly expect to be lifelong users of the Castor Oil Pack, we're more interested in knowing about your experiences with this outstanding therapy. If you have information on how you use these products and would like to see your information included in our next edition, please let us know. You can call us at 800-269-2502, or email us at info@baar.com. You can also write to us at Baar Products, PO Box 60, Downingtown, PA 19335.

As always, we look forward to hearing from you!

Bruce Baar MS, ND
Kathy Baar RDH, BS

Notes

_____

_____

_____

_____

_____

_____

_____

_____

_____

_____

_____

_____

_____

_____

_____

_____

_____

Afterword

This book was completed with the help of our customers and our staff.

Please feel free to call or write to us with any questions as you get started – and with your comments once you've completed several applications. As always, we look forward to hearing from you!

Baar Products
PO Box 60
Downingtown, PA 19335

call us:
800-269-2502

or email us:
info@baar.com

48590053R00031

Made in the USA
Charleston, SC
06 November 2015